"I have known Sally Faith for more than thirty-five years, and it doesn't surprise me that she would write such a candid book about her struggles with dementia to benefit others. This is an extension of her long-time commitment to serve others as she takes this opportunity to help individuals and families alike who are dealing with life-altering loss of memory. Thank you, Sally. You are an inspiration!"

—Steve Ehlmann

Saint Charles County Executive

"Sally Faith has discovered the gifts that God gave her and uses them to make a difference in the lives of others. Sally lights up a room whenever she enters and shares her warmth, grace, and contagious joy while she is there. I may not remember the last time I saw Sally, but I will always remember how she made me feel.

Thank you for writing this book, Sally, and for sharing your journey and attitude with others. I am honored that you call me your friend."

—Nancy Young

Leader, Alzheimer's Group

"Sally's recollection of her early diagnosis had to be very therapeutic for her, as it would be for others. Removing her fears early was smart and good advice for anyone facing this news."

—Ann Hazelwood, Author

"Sally has been an outstanding public servant and continues giving back to the community she loves by offering first-hand experience to others with this book."

—Randy Schilling
Founder, OPO Startups

"As with everything Sally tackles, she has faced her diagnosis with determination, directness, and good humor. I've had the gift of Sally's friendship for over thirty years; her book is a gift to all of us."

—Phyllis Schnieder

"Sally and I had an afternoon visit planned. It just so happened to be the day after her diagnosis. She shared her news but didn't have a plan for sharing the news of her early dementia with others. The unknowns of her future were uncomfortable for both of us as we sat in her garden.

When Sally decided to write this book, it offered her the freedom to manage her fears about her future while being of service to others. *I'm Losing My Memory; I'm NOT Losing My Mind* has brought out the politician in Sally. Now she uses her passion for service to tell her story, so others will learn from her journey of early dementia. I cannot think of a better advocate!

—Denise Liebel

President & CEO,

United Services for Children

"Sally Faith is a genuinely kind and caring person, and indeed a fun-loving extrovert! She is also appropriately named. She exudes energy, concern, friendliness, and a can-do attitude. It appears that her positive attitude, as evidenced by her enlightening book, serves her well while dealing with her dementia diagnosis. Her attitude is a source of personal strength that should inspire others. At her core, in addition to her strong faith, is Sally's great strength is her lifelong commitment to serving others. At a time when she could justifiably feel sorry for herself, she remains focused on finding ways to continue serving others . . . including the writing of this courageous book . . . a true act of faith!!"

—Jenny and Greg VanWyk, Kilwins

"Thank you, Sally, for having the courage to share your experiences and your fears as a community leader diagnosed with early dementia. As a public servant, it's not always easy to share personal challenges. As an individual who has personally lost friends and loved ones to Alzheimer's, your quick-read book helped me to better understand what they and their caregivers may have also experienced. I appreciate your willingness to be open to help others recently diagnosed who may be experiencing similar feelings and fears. This book lets them know they are not alone."

—Scott Tate
President & CEO,
Saint Charles Regional Chamber

"By sharing her diagnosis, Sally Faith has helped me understand the fears, anxieties, and frustrations with living with early dementia. The fear of being isolated, a burden, and the loss of control can be overwhelming. But as leader and a problem solver, Sally shares how to take back control and develop a plan. With her positive attitude and her plan, she will live on her own terms."

—Rose Wells

"What a wonderful story—the fears, pain, frustrations, and truths about dealing personally with a scary diagnosis. Sally is a tough cookie and is always pushing forward. I am proud to call her a friend. Share this book with someone you know who is dealing with dementia or is a caregiver!"

—Mark A Hollander
Executive Director / Vision St Charles
County Leadership

"I've had the pleasure of knowing Sally Faith for over twenty years. Her genuine gift of always being there to guide, support, and encourage others was an extraordinarily admirable quality. Now, when she could have kept to herself and navigated this disease in silence, she once again put herself out where the community might benefit from this new experience and knowledge.

—April Moxley

Owner of April's on Main

I'm Losing My Memory; I'm NOT Losing My Mind

I'm Losing My Memory;
I'm NOT Losing My Mind

A Frank Perspective about Living with Early Dementia

Sally Faith

Stonebrook Publishing
Saint Louis, Missouri

A STONEBROOK PUBLISHING BOOK
©2022 Sally Faith

This book was guided in development and
edited by Nancy L. Erickson, The Book Professor®
TheBookProfessor.com

Library of Congress Control Number: 2022909566

ISBN: 978-1-955711-15-9

www.stonebrookpublishing.net

Contents

1. The Unwelcome Truth 1

2. Tell the World 13

3. Paralyzing Fears — and Their Remedies . . .23

    Fear 1: Family History 26

    Fear 2: I'm Afraid of a Rapid Decline 36

    Fear 3: I'm Afraid of Losing My
               Independence. 52

    Fear 4: I'm Worried about the
               Cost of Long-Term Care 79

    Fear 5: I'm Grieving over Losing
               My Memory. 84

    Fear 6: I'm Embarrassed about
               the Changes 88

    Fear 7: I Don't Want to Be Isolated 96

4. A Son's Perspective on Caregiving 107

5. In Closing 115

About the Author 117

1

The Unwelcome Truth

I KNEW SOMETHING was wrong, but I didn't know what it was or who to ask for help. I was forgetting the names of decades-old dear friends. I couldn't come up with the word I wanted to say. I couldn't remember what I was supposed to do that day, and worse, I was losing my ability to figure it out. But I kept it to myself. Surely these were minor things that were part of the normal aging process.

And then things changed. My son, Howard, called and asked if he could stop by one Saturday. It was a beautiful, warm, breezy summer day. I'd been sitting on my patio reading a book and enjoying the waterfall and the breeze. Birds flew into the arborvitaes before their bath. They flapped their wings several times, then jumped into the waterfall for a drink. I was looking forward to seeing Howard.

We sat down and Howard told me about the phone calls he'd received from a couple of my girlfriends. They'd seen some changes and were concerned about me. Of course, he didn't mention their names.

"They think you're depressed, Mom, and that you might need some help."

"I'm not depressed," I answered. "That's ridiculous. I'm fine."

"Actually, Mary and I have noticed some changes too," he said.

Every week, I saw Howard and his wife for lunch on Sundays. Had they been evaluating me during our weekly time together?

"We think your friends have a good point, Mom," Howard continued. "Something's off. I think we need to find out what's going on."

Howard's comments really surprised me—infuriated me, to tell the truth—but I said nothing. I was shocked. And here's something you should know about me: I never say nothing. I've been a politician for most of my life, and you know we love to talk. Sometimes we talk when we don't have anything to say, but I was stunned into silence. I was furious that my friends had called my son instead of me. It wasn't Howard's fault that they'd put him in this position, so I tried to remain calm because I didn't want to blame him.

"Okay," I said. "I guess I'll make an appointment with Dr. Kramer, but I'd like you to be there with me," I said. "Will you come?"

I'd been a patient of Dr. Daniel Kramer's for many years, and I trusted him. He'd done all my annual checkups and had all my medical information. I wanted Howard to go with me, so we'd hear and see the same thing at the same time. Two heads are better than one, right? I quickly got an appointment, and I made sure they knew that Howard would be there.

We sat down, and I said, "I'm here because my friends called Howard, not me, and they think I'm having problems."

"Well, Sally, you have some very good friends. You should thank them," Dr. Kramer said.

That's not what I expected or wanted to hear. I was furious that people had gone behind my back and had talked to my son.

Dr. Kramer gave me some simple cognitive skill tests, and when I couldn't remember five items from one moment to the next, I was told I had signs of early dementia. How could that be? I remembered the name of the president. How could I have dementia? I got very quiet.

"Tell me," Dr. Kramer said. "Is there any history of dementia in your family?"

"My mother died of Alzheimer's fifteen years ago," I answered.

"And how old was she?" he asked.

"Seventy-four," I said.

"Sally, if she died when she was only seventy-four, then she must have had early dementia too."

I didn't like that. I didn't want to be there. I didn't want to be having this conversation, but I was stuck for the time being and wanted to quickly wrap up this visit.

"So what do I do now?" I asked.

"Let me give you a couple names of some neurologists. I suggest you see at least one of them for a second opinion. That's your next step," he said.

Howard and I went back to my house, and I sat on my swing. I was stone-cold quiet.

"You seem pretty calm, Mom," Howard said.

"I don't have anything to say," I murmured. And I didn't. What do you say when you've just been told that you're losing your mind?

A couple weeks later, Howard and I went to see Dr. Min Pan, a neurologist. I liked her. She was up front and direct. She asked about my family history, tested my memory, and asked me questions about the events of the current year. She also watched how I walked.

"You need to concentrate on your feet when you walk," she said. "Walk like this: heel, toe, heel, toe."

So now I couldn't walk right either? I wondered what that meant.

After the evaluation was complete, Dr. Min Pan addressed Howard and me.

"Sally, I agree with Dr. Kramer. You have early dementia," she said. "There's medication that could potentially slow it down, but it's not curable. It will progress and get worse over time. I'm very sorry."

Another bombshell. Medication could only maybe slow it down—but not fix it? I was devastated. I wanted to wrap my head around what I was hearing, but all I heard was bad news. Where was the hope in this diagnosis? What would my future look like?

So many questions swirled in my mind, but again, I was silent. I needed to process this devastating news.

And daily medication? All my life, I'd taken no more than one pill per day. I didn't want to become a walking pharmacy.

It was hard to adjust to this news, and finding a new direction wasn't easy. But I'm here to tell you that I did overcome, and I have moved forward. I've always moved forward at different times in my life, and I was determined to do so now.

Here's what I know: We have dementia and cannot change that. IT'S OKAY.

So why did I write this book? I want to share what I'm learning about having early dementia and navigating those challenges to provide hope if you've recently received the same diagnosis. Early dementia can't be kept a secret. Talking openly about my life

> IT WAS HARD TO ADJUST TO THIS NEWS, AND FINDING A NEW DIRECTION WASN'T EASY. BUT I'M HERE TO TELL YOU THAT I DID OVERCOME, AND I HAVE MOVED FORWARD.

experiences helps me as well as you. The purpose of this book is to offer hope and help if you've been diagnosed with dementia and to show you how to develop a positive mindset as you progress through the stages of this illness.

Follow me; I'll show you how I've navigated these waters and kept my dignity intact and my humor in place. We have dementia and cannot change that. IT'S OKAY!

2

Tell the World

I'VE ALWAYS BEEN a high-energy, involved person, and I love being out and about meeting people and listening to their stories, their joys, and their concerns. And my career gave me plenty of opportunities to do that.

While I was working, I held several elected positions. I was always out in the public, reaching out and talking to individuals. I gave lectures and speeches throughout the communities. My first elected office was to the First Community College of Saint Charles County. I was elected to its Board of Trustees in April 1986. I served there until November of 1994. I was elected and sworn into the Saint Charles County Council and served from January 1995 to December 2004. I served in the Missouri House of Representatives for four two-year terms starting January 2005 to April 2011. I gave up my seat in April 2011, when I was elected as Mayor of the City of Saint Charles, Missouri, and I served two four-year terms. I retired on

June 1, 2019, at the age of seventy-four—the same age that my mother was when she died.

As a politician, I've always had the gift of gab. But I wasn't sure if I should talk about having early dementia. Should I keep it a secret? Did I have to hide out to conceal it from the public that I'd grown to love? In discussions with some of my friends, I told them I didn't

> BUT I WASN'T SURE IF I SHOULD TALK ABOUT HAVING EARLY DEMENTIA. SHOULD I KEEP IT A SECRET?

know how to go forward. I wondered if I should tell anyone about it until I had more information.

One friend said, "Don't tell anyone. People would look at you differently and will avoid you." I certainly didn't want that to happen. But after much thought, I decided that I wanted to be in control of my story and my life, and I wanted to be in control of how my story was told. And, clearly, people had already noticed that I was different. I had early dementia, and that was okay. I hadn't done anything to be ashamed of, so I wasn't going to live my life in shame. I thought it would be best to take the bull by the horns and take control of my story.

But what do you say? "Oh! By the way, I have early dementia. Pass the coffee."

Who would I tell and not tell? How would I tell them? After much contemplation, I came up with a plan. My first outreach to tell others was around Christmastime. Most people knew I was retired, and they would ask, "What are you doing now?"

I answered, "I'm writing a book."

"Really? What's it about?" they'd say.

And then came my reveal. "I was told I have early dementia, and I'm writing about my challenges."

Those poor folks. That's when they stopped asking questions. I understood that they didn't know what to say after that. But I was trying to hold my ground and hang on to my story. And it worked out perfectly. Time after time, when people asked me what involved me now, I told them the same thing: I'm writing a book about having early dementia. And it became easier and easier for me to say it and also easier for my friends and associates to hear it.

When I decided to be open about my early dementia, a weight was lifted off my shoulders. I didn't want to pretend, I didn't want to hide, I didn't want to avoid people, and I didn't want to make excuses for myself. Now I don't have to. And the grace and support I've received have been overwhelming.

And everyone was curious about the book—this book. Talking about this book gave us an entry into a meaningful conversation. This gave my friends permission to talk about what I was experiencing and for me to share how they could help. They often asked why I was writing the book.

"I want to write about my experiences, so others who have dementia will know what to expect, but also so their friends and caregivers will know how to talk to them. We're still here. Yes, we have dementia, but we want to be included and respected. We want to participate in a full life. We don't want anyone to be afraid of us or to be afraid they'll say the wrong thing," I'd say.

And that discussion would lead to another, more detailed account of what I faced in the future.

"I have dementia, and I'm going to lose my short-term memory and eventually some long-term memory. But I'm still me, and I'm still your friend. It's a progressive brain disease. There's no treatment plan, and there's no cure. But my soul and heart are still inside."

My point is this: You don't have anything to be ashamed of. You have no reason to hide. Trust that the people who know and love you want to be included in this part of your life.

Yes, we have dementia, but that's okay! By this age, everyone has something, and nobody feels the need to be private about their hip replacement, their sore knees, or even their prostate cancer. Aging bodies have issues. This one is yours.

You'll lose a lot more than your memory if you lose contact with others, so tell people what's happening and keep those relationships alive.

> MY POINT IS THIS: YOU DON'T HAVE ANYTHING TO BE ASHAMED OF. YOU HAVE NO REASON TO HIDE.

Yes, we have early dementia, and that's okay!

3

Paralyzing Fears — and Their Remedies

OF COURSE, DEMENTIA feels serious, and I suppose it is. A lot of things are changing with me, and even more changes will come in the future. But as a problem solver, I decided that the best thing to do was to adopt a positive attitude and to get out ahead of it, so I could maintain as much control of my life as possible for as long as possible.

The first thing we must all do is face the diagnosis. What the doctor told you is not a mistake. You and I have dementia, and that's okay. It's up to us to decide how we're going to handle our lives going forward. I decided from the start that I didn't want to become a burden to my family—to my son, who is an only child—and I decided that I'd do whatever needed to be done to avoid that.

The second thing I had to do was face my fears. Of course, this scares me! Of course, I feel that rise of panic from time to time. I've always treasured my mind, my quick wit, my problem-solving abilities, and my memory! Of course, I don't want to lose those things. But since that's what will happen eventually (and you know there's no way to predict how quickly the decline will come), I decided I would do *now* the things I probably wouldn't be able to do later.

> THE FIRST THING WE MUST ALL DO IS FACE THE DIAGNOSIS. NO, WHAT THE DOCTOR TOLD YOU IS NOT A MISTAKE. YOU AND I HAVE DEMENTIA, AND THAT'S OKAY.

In fact, I had a lot of fears, and I bet you do too. In fact, I'm certain we have some of the same fears. But I decided early on to face them head-on, so I could live my life to the fullest.

Fear 1: Family History

How long do I have? No one knows. My mother, Florence Killian, passed away in December of 2000 at Saint Peter's Manor Nursing Home of Alzheimer's at age 74. So, I've already outlived her. And her story is different from mine, even though we arrived at the same diagnosis.

My mother was living near Pevely, Missouri, when she had a stroke. I had to quickly become educated about Medicare, assisted living, and skilled nursing, and I needed to find a nursing home close by—all within a week's time. When she was released from the hospital, she moved into a nursing home in Pevely. My thought was that she had friends in Pevely who would come visit her, and her church was nearby, so they'd be involved in her care. But I was wrong. She wasn't receiving the visitors I thought she would have, and as time went by, it became more and more difficult for me to get from Saint Charles to Pevely during rush hour. Spending time with her on a regular basis was practically impossible. So, I decided to move her near me to Saint Peters, where

I could get to her quickly and be there frequently.

It's important to make it as easy as possible for the caregiver to support the person they're responsible for. And it's much easier if they are nearby. Visiting frequently, being her advocate, and attending meetings at the nursing home were important to me, and Saint Peters Manor was located between the college where I worked and my home. It was convenient for me to stop by without having a routine to follow. My mother lived there for seven years.

I loved to play the piano in the dining area for the residents. I'd play familiar songs, and they would sing along. During the holidays, I decorated Mom's room, and on Christmas morning, I went by and played Christmas songs, so we could sing and celebrate.

> IT'S IMPORTANT TO MAKE IT AS EASY AS POSSIBLE FOR THE CAREGIVER TO SUPPORT THE PERSON THEY'RE RESPONSIBLE FOR.

But we couldn't stop her decline.

One time, her brothers came to visit her. Tommy was from Louisiana, and Bob was from California. Tommy drove to California to pick up Bob, and they both rode together to Saint Charles to visit her. Mother sat there and looked at them, listening. But she had no idea who they were. Oddly enough, she remembered other relatives she hadn't seen in a lifetime, but not them. And before she died, she told me a shocking story.

On my way to work one day, I stopped by to check on her. When I walked into her room, she said, "You have a brother one year younger than you, and I put him up for adoption."

What? That didn't make sense. I'd always been an only child. So, my first question was, *Is she clear of mind?* I had to verify whether this bombshell was true, so I sent her older sister a letter and told her what my mother had said.

My aunt wrote back, "You have a good life. Forget about it."

I had no idea how to find out if I had a brother out there. But my brother's adoptive parents had given him the information about his adoption and what they knew about his biological family. His oldest child searched on the internet to find his paternal grandmother. He discovered where Mom's family was and that she also had a daughter—me. My brother's name is Terry.

He then contacted my uncle Tommy in Louisiana to see if I would like to have Terry call me, and Tommy told me about the phone call.

"Sally, I got a call from your nephew who said that his father is your brother and that he was adopted at birth. Are you okay with him calling you?"

It was snowing that day in Saint Charles. My mother had passed away six months earlier, and I was missing her. Her decline and ultimate death had been hard to witness. She was once a strong, independent woman, but in the end, she was almost unrecognizable. She wasn't the mother I'd grown up with. I told my uncle that I'd love to get together with my brother.

When Terry called, he sounded normal. We talked about our families for a while and then about our mother. I told him I was running for the Missouri House of Representatives.

"I bet you're a Republican," he said.

"And I bet you're a Democrat!"

We hit it off on the phone and made plans for him and his son to visit Saint Charles. Waiting for them at the Saint Louis airport, I held a photo of both of them. I was a nervous wreck, so to cope, I kept eating chocolate! It was summertime, and the airport was crowded with people. I strained to search for them in the crowd, then finally recognized them. I gave them a big hug and took them out for dinner in Saint Charles.

"What was she like?" Terry asked about our mother.

"Well, she was many things," I said, "and she was different at different points in her life." I wanted to concentrate on her good years, her vibrant years.

"Did you know about me?" Terry asked.

"No. I always thought I was an only child. Mother only told me about you a short while before she died. And even then, I couldn't be sure it was true because she had fallen so far into her dementia. If I'd known about you, Terry, I would have found you before now."

After dinner, I gave them a tour of Saint Charles and showed them where Mother and

I had lived and where she was buried. Terry asked if he could have some private time to talk to his mother. I respected that request.

Before Terry and his son left town, I invited them to visit my church. I played the piano at Saint Charles Church of God, and that week, the sermon was about families. When my mother passed away, I felt totally, utterly alone. And when I found out that I had a brother, I was delighted. I had gained a brother, a sister-in-law, two nephews, and one niece, who all live in California. This made me very happy. My brother and nephew flew back to San Francisco later that day, and we have stayed in touch since then.

But the fact of my mother's history with dementia—and that she'd lived in a care facility for seven years—weighed on me. I didn't want to be like that. I didn't want to lose my mind. I didn't want to lose myself.

Fear 2: I'm Afraid of a Rapid Decline

I didn't know what to expect with dementia. I was afraid I'd forget my friends right away. I couldn't bear to think that I wouldn't recognize my friends and family. But that's *end-stage dementia*, not early stage.

As the mayor of Saint Charles, I always met people—our citizens—out on the street and about in public. My memory was razor sharp. I knew who they were, could connect a face with a name, and knew the ins and outs of the issues they wanted to talk about. I also either knew the answer to their questions or knew who could help them.

I'd always thought it was funny when people would tell me that they'd walked into the bedroom and couldn't remember why they were there. *That's odd,* I thought. *I'm never going to be that way.*

Now it's not so funny.

My memory has always been important to me. I know a lot of people, and it's important to recognize and communicate with others. I'm an extrovert. And if I couldn't communicate, I'd be all alone, and that's not what I wanted. I love people, and I reach out to them. To not be able to do that or to forget my connections was a frightful prospect. I was afraid that I wouldn't be me if I lost that.

Nobody knows how quickly or how slowly my dementia—or yours—will progress. But I know the decline is coming. And I've been concerned that it will happen quickly. Will there be enough money? Will I have the finances to support myself? Will I have the strength and energy to keep going? Will I be prepared if my decline happens quickly, and will I be prepared if it *doesn't* happen quickly?

In a situation like this, you have to think about your money. I was afraid I wouldn't be financially able to do what I wanted

> NOBODY KNOWS HOW QUICKLY OR HOW SLOWLY MY DEMENTIA— OR YOURS—WILL PROGRESS. BUT I KNOW THE DECLINE IS COMING.

to do. Worse yet, I didn't really know what I wanted! Would I lose my house? That thought scared me.

I decided I needed to know the facts, so I could make decisions for myself while I could still make decisions. My son, Howard, was so helpful in this respect. He helped me establish clear financial practices, and he evaluated my investments, so I could see that I had what I needed to take care of myself. That was such a relief. Now I know what I have, and I love feeling financially responsible for myself.

Howard and I sit down together to work on my finances every week. He comes by after work one night a week, and we talk about my finances, where the money is spent, and how the budget looks. We don't agree on every-thing, but we talk through how I'm spending my money. This takes the pressure off my son because we're approaching this together. He has power of attorney over everything, but he won't exercise it until I can no longer make decisions for myself, and as long as we keep the communication going, I'll be in charge of my money.

This process has relieved me of the fear of a rapid decline. Week by week, I know how I'm doing financially, and I know that I can still handle my finances with Howard's help. He continues to empower me this way, and I so appreciate it.

Managing my medications was another matter. My doctor prescribed meds to slow the progression of my dementia, and I also take B12 and D3 supplements. But they only work if I take them as prescribed!

My first problem was that I couldn't remember if I'd taken my pills. Was this a sign that I was getting worse? I'd be positive that I'd taken them, but then I'd see them sitting there in the pill box. The confusion around taking my medicine was crippling at times. I panicked when I discovered I hadn't taken it.

Taking multiple medications throughout the day was confusing because I'd never had to do that before. I had to know exactly what medication to take and when to take it. I wanted this to be my responsibility, but I was having problems keeping track of these things.

I knew I was smart enough to figure out the pills. *I'm an intelligent person,* I thought. *Why can't I do this?* It was like when I decided to learn to play golf when Howard was playing golf too. I thought it would be a good way for the two of us to spend time together. When I got out on the course, I thought, *I should be able to do this.* But I was terrible at it, and I was embarrassed. But I kept at it and finally figured it out. The pills were just like that.

I discussed it with Howard, and he suggested I use a pill box. Using a weekly pillbox for morning and evening medications helped me to keep track of my meds, and it gave me confidence.

But there's more to it than simply loading up a pillbox every week. When I pick up a prescription, I always verify that I've got the right meds at the correct strength. I learned this the hard way when the wrong strength was given to me one time, so I now closely check what I receive. As I have even more meds, I'm more determined to closely watch and verify. If it doesn't look right, I call the prescribing doctor to verify it.

Howard also helped me by setting my cell phone alert to go off at 7:00 a.m. and

6:00 p.m. to remind me to take my pills. Managing my medications is going much better now. It's not perfect every day, but it's much better. The last thing I want to do is forget to take the medication that could slow my decline!

I'd also heard that there were other fun things I could do to help preserve my memory. I've always been a social person, and I intend to keep up with my friends and activities. Being out and about and meeting with people keeps you active, and being active is a deterrent to decline. I sit down every week to plan lunch outings with friends, and I attend my book club every month.

And I've learned that I can exercise my brain by learning to play chess. In fact, I found out that the Saint Louis chess club has gatherings for first-time female players, and I plan to attend those. And I've discovered the *Brain Games - Find the Cat Challenge* book, which is a bit like the *Where's Waldo?* books. Kind of simplistic but fun! Of course, working on crossword puzzles has long been established as a way to exercise the brain.

> I'D ALSO HEARD THAT THERE WERE OTHER FUN THINGS I COULD DO TO HELP PRESERVE MY MEMORY.

I've always been an avid reader, and because I've stayed curious, I read a lot. I read the daily newspaper, the *Business Journal*, the free grocery store papers, and, of course, books. I'm delighted that I can still comprehend what I'm reading. If I keep up this practice, I believe I'll preserve this part of my cognition.

I've met people who no longer read books because they don't understand what the words say. I had no idea this could happen. I thought that I'd always be able to read, retain, and understand what I'd read, but I found out that sometimes people with dementia lose the ability to read.

A friend of mine said, "You like golf. Do you want this book?'

I really didn't want the book and told him so.

"Well, I can't read anymore because I don't understand or remember what it says. My family keeps giving me books, and I don't know how to tell them I can't read them anymore."

This surprised me because this man seemed perfectly capable of carrying on a conversation. And he played golf, so it seemed like a book about golf would be a good choice for him. I didn't see any signs of dementia because he was so active.

Will this happen to me? At what stage does this occur? I read a lot—all the time, in fact. I may be experiencing advanced grief over the possibility of losing this tool and pleasure in my life, but will I even know when it happens? My friend didn't seem bothered that he couldn't read anymore. Since I don't know what's going to happen in the future, I think I'll just concentrate on today.

Another way to stretch my brain capacity is to use my nondominant hand in routine tasks. I'm right-handed, so when I brush my teeth, eat meals, or wash out the kitchen sink, I frequently test myself by using my left hand. It's not easy—and I don't really like it—but I can practically feel my brain synapses growing and glowing.

The first good news I heard about my condition was that dementia wouldn't change my ability to play the piano and remember words to songs. My lifelong love of music brings me so much pleasure. I still study the piano and perform whenever I can. My goal is to be one hundred years old and still going!

My goal is to stay active and not let my world

> THE FIRST GOOD NEWS I HEARD ABOUT MY CONDITION WAS THAT DEMENTIA WOULDN'T CHANGE MY ABILITY TO PLAY THE PIANO AND REMEMBER WORDS TO SONGS.

shrink. I'm worried that someday I'll withdraw from people and friends, so I work every day to put myself out there. It's important that I make contact with my friends and family, but I have to reach out to them. I don't sit around waiting for them to reach out to me.

And what about a bucket list? Are there things I want to do before I can no longer do them? Of course! I want to have enough time to read the books that I want, to play the music I want to play, to reach out to new people, to support my friends, to ride a train across the northern part of the United States.

But the truth is that you only need a bucket list if you haven't been doing the things you want to do all along. I was so busy in my working and political life that I didn't have the time to concentrate on my family and friends. Now I want to focus on them. And that's just about all I want to do.

Fear 3: I'm Afraid of Losing My Independence

Hey, I've been on my own for decades, and one of the things I prize the most is my independence. I've lived on my own, made decisions on my own, and have flourished on my own for so long that the prospect of becoming weak and dependent on someone else—anyone else—is not only foreign, but also frightening.

I decided early on that it's important for me to take care of myself. Don't hand your life over to others, to caregivers. We should help our caregivers, but not resign to them. Maintain your adulthood as long as possible, rather than becoming a child in your later years. You're capable of many things, and your life has proven that.

> I DECIDED EARLY ON THAT IT'S IMPORTANT FOR ME TO TAKE CARE OF MYSELF. DON'T HAND YOUR LIFE OVER TO OTHERS, TO CAREGIVERS.

But that doesn't mean you can't preserve a childlike curiosity and penchant for fun. There are some interesting ways to revert to your youth without becoming a dependent child. For example, just last month, I was in a fashion show at the Foundry in Saint Charles, Missouri, for men and women who are fifty-five years and older. The fun part was getting together with the organizers and getting dressed for the event in clothes that I didn't own but looked like they were made just for me. They did my hair, my makeup, and provided jewelry and other accessories. I looked like a million bucks! And when I strutted down the runway, there was raving applause. Now *that* was fun!

Of course, almost every aging person hates the idea of losing their independence. But for dementia patients, it's a looming reality that has a sharp bite.

For me, independence means that I can come and go, do what I want, and make my own decisions without having to involve others. But I know that's a reality for only a short time, so like with everything else, I decided to get out ahead of it and decide now what I wanted for my future.

The most pressing factor was my living arrangement. It seemed clear that I wouldn't be able to live alone in my house forever, so my first thought was to stay at home as long as I could by taking advantage of home care services. So I contacted a few agencies, but then I thought, *Sally, aren't you just delaying the inevitable? Shouldn't you figure out a long-term solution?*

That's when I started making appointments to tour senior care facilities to gather details and information about rooms, costs, etc. Since it was inevitable that I was going to move, I wanted to be in charge of where I went. It was important that my son and I agreed on where I would live, and we toured local facilities together.

Yes, I was anxious, scared, and apprehensive about moving into a place that would eventually provide me with memory care. Making a plan for your future is a great idea, but it's also very painful. It can be very overwhelming. But it's also an expression of my independence, and that's important to me.

YES, I WAS ANXIOUS, SCARED, AND APPREHENSIVE ABOUT MOVING INTO A MEMORY CARE UNIT. . . . BUT IT'S ALSO AN EXPRESSION OF MY INDEPENDENCE. AND THAT'S IMPORTANT TO ME.

My friend, Nancy, invited me to tour Lake Saint Charles Senior Living. We scheduled a lunch date there to view the facility, and I explained that when I was mayor of Saint Charles, I'd attended an annual Veterans Day program there. I was already familiar with the location, but I hadn't thought about the possibility of living there.

As I walked up the front sidewalk and into the building, I knew this was where I wanted to move. It just felt right. I had lunch with Nancy, but I didn't say anything to anyone until the next day.

"Howard, I was at the Lake Saint Charles Senior Living Center yesterday, and I had an overwhelming feeling that it's the right place for me. That's where I want to move."

He was surprised. We'd done a lot of facility touring together, and in fact, I'd already made future arrangements to move somewhere else.

"Are you certain?" he asked.

"I am. And I want to move there as soon as possible. I want to be able to make the decisions about what to take from my house to my apartment while I have the clear mind to decide those things for myself."

I didn't want someone else to decide where I'd go and what I'd take when I moved from my lovely home. No guilt. No regrets. I was at peace with my decision.

Howard was relieved that the decision had been made. On October 2, 2021, about forty-five days later, I moved to Lake Saint Charles Independent Living.

Looking to the future, I'm prepared to have the everyday things I need to enjoy the time that I have left. Time to write, read, enjoy friends, and do spur-of-the-moment fun things just for me. My family and I no longer have to worry about falling, security, changing my sheets, maintaining the lawn, grocery shopping, house maintenance, and paying the bills. Fortunately, my lovely home will stay in my family because my grandson purchased it from me.

My new location is perfectly situated near stores, restaurants, doctors, the post office, my church, and my friends. I love my new home because it gives me another outlet for being social.

I want the personal contact that community living provides; I know I need that. Of course, there are people here who I don't know by name—because I can't remember their names—and I talk to everyone I pass to continue my connection with people. I eat at a table with three other women, and I've enjoyed getting to know them.

But here's the kicker: I've already touched the lives of people in this facility by listening to them and caring about them. I can actually reach more people here, and I can make them feel significant.

Do you know what those of us with dementia are most afraid of? We're afraid of fading away, of becoming ghostlike. I won't let that happen to the people around me. I want to know that I'm not disappearing and that they aren't either. That's what I strive for in our community.

And I get to step in and step out because I have my own car, which most of the other residents don't have. Driving is important to me. It's more than a symbol of independence; it's my freedom!

I don't drive at night, but that doesn't mean I'm willing to miss out on evening entertainment. Not long ago, I was invited to a birthday party that was at night, so I called someone and asked if I could ride with them. That guy didn't like to drive at night either, so I phoned someone else. I didn't give up, and I went to the party.

But here's the thing: it was the first time I'd ever asked anyone for a ride, and I really didn't like doing that. But I'm not going to let that stop me from participating in life. No, I don't want to ask people for rides too often, but when I need to, I will. I have to set aside my pride and ego and ask for the help I need. That's one aspect of my new independence.

Of course, I want to keep driving as long as I can. Sometimes I drive Howard places, and I know he's monitoring my driving. He probably should. We've talked about when it might be time for me to give up the keys because that's one more thing that's inevitable. That time is definitely coming. It's just not today.

"When you decide that it's time for me to stop driving, we'll have that discussion, and I'll listen to you," I told him.

I don't want something drastic to happen, and I don't want to hurt anyone, so I have plans for how I'll get around when I can no longer drive.

Over my years as a public servant, I'd been asked to join many organizations as a member of their board of directors, and one of them was ITN Gateway, a ride service that provides "dignified transportation for seniors." Its mission is to provide a community-based and community-supported, economically viable, and consumer-oriented, quality transportation service for seniors and visually impaired adults. I'm proud to say that I helped start this organization.

In a nutshell, volunteers drive older people where they need to go, such as doctor visits, appointments, shopping, etc. They pick you up and take you home. There's no cash involved because it's a membership basis. You put money in your account every month, and you don't have to fumble with cash on the day you need a ride.

When we were forming this service for seniors, I never thought I'd be a customer. For now, I only use it when I don't want to drive someplace myself. As long as I make a reservation in advance, I know I'll have a ride. And I know the day will come when ITN Gateway is my primary means of transportation. In fact, I'm planning on it. My concern about giving up my independence is overshadowed by my determination to keep going.

Here are some of the things I do to continue living as an independent adult:

- Managing my calendar. Because I don't want to miss anything that I've committed to doing, I've started keeping track of my life on a large calendar. I was starting to put things in the wrong box, which caused me to miss out on things. I still get confused, so I have to fully focus on putting items in the correct box for that day. I worked out a system

where I go back and review my
calendar several times a day to make
sure that I show up at the right
place at the right time on the right
date. I never had a problem with
this before, but I've compensated by
sticking to what's on paper and not
relying on my memory.

I check my calendar frequently
during the day, and I check and
recheck it. I verify where I'm supposed to go and what I'm supposed
to be doing. And I make plans fur-
ther ahead than I used to. Making
plans helps me feel like I'm going to

be here in the future. If I don't plan ahead, it's like I'm giving up and accepting that I might not be here someday.

I'm getting more detailed as I deal with dementia. It's important for me to check and verify everything. Details are more important to me now than ever.

- Organizing. When I see something I might need to use or do in the future, I put it in a specific place, so I'll know where it is when I need it. I hate to lose something or redo something, so I make sure I know where everything is. Being organized helps my son and me communicate during our weekly meetings.

He'll say, "Do you have this and this?" and I say, "It's here some-where, and I'll have it the next time you come." Being organized helps me not to panic.

- In the kitchen. I don't cook, and I don't want to. But I do use the cof-fee pot. Sometimes I put the coffee in there and forget to put water in, so when I push the button, nothing happens. So I put water in it. And one time, I put in the water and forgot to put the cup under it! So now, when I start making coffee, I open the cupboard door, which makes me realize there's more to do—like get a cup!

- Keeping track of items. When I set something down, like my glasses, I lay them on something white, so I can see them. Then I look at them for a moment to help me remember where I put them. My intention is to always lay them in the same spot so I don't have to look for them.

Of course, this applies to other items too.

- Grooming. I put the shampoo in the same place every time or else I'll put conditioner on my hair instead of shampoo! I make sure the shampoo is first in line and the conditioner second. And I leave my makeup in the same spot, so I don't have to hunt for the individual pieces.

  Grooming is important to me, and I want to start wearing earrings again. It's important not to start giving up things. For example, I love having my nails look nice. And here's an example of how important it is to me: At my current home, they were bringing in White Castle for the residents, and we could sign up to get some, which I did. But then my friend who does my nails called and said she could take me that morning—and that was my priority. I was a little late for lunch, but I got my nails done.

- Clothing. I separated all my clothes into colors, so I can find them easily and match my outfits.

- Remembering things. When I think of something, I do it right then because if I don't, I'll forget. Make a phone call, write a note, pick up something—I DO IT NOW. I don't want to forget it.

  For a while, I was writing things down, but then I didn't go back and look at the piece of paper. Putting it on paper took it off my mind, so I never thought about it again. Clearly, that wasn't working. So now I do things immediately.

- Phone calls. I make a list of who I want to call and the reason for the call. Then I write down the phone number so that when I'm ready to make calls, I have all the information I need.

- Grocery shopping. I make a grocery list that has three columns across the top: What I'd like to get / What I need / What I can afford. I have a weekly budget, and I don't want to overspend. I'm very conscious of my money because, if I lose control of my spending, that's an indication to my son that I can't handle my life, and I don't want that.

- Keeping routines. I've started going to stretching classes where I live. I have breakfast at 7:30, and I know that with dementia, it's important to keep your same routine. I'm getting up, eating, coming back up, and doing my day. I'm making contact with other people, which is good every day.

- Rut busters. It's easy to get into a rut, and although people with dementia benefit from routine, we need to continue to develop our brain capacity. Here are some things I like to do to mix it up.

o In my community living, I don't go in the same door as I go out.

o I frequently move things around in my apartment—on purpose. I don't want to see the same things every day FOR THE REST OF MY LIFE. For years, I've put all my pocket change into a big pot. Yesterday, I took out all the change and sorted it. Then I got other dishes for each type of coin.

o When I drive, I try to take a different route. Driving the same way each time is developing a rut.

o I go to a different grocery store from time to time. I may not like that store, but I go there to mix things up and break the routine. That makes me relearn my life. It's stimulating.

o Where I live, there are different ways to go to the elevator, and I

take a different route each time.
It helps me connect the different
dots. There's more than one way
to do things!

As long as I do these things, I'm making
the choice to exercise my independence. And
that feels good.

Fear 4: I'm Worried about the Cost of Long-Term Care

Let's face it. Few of us with dementia will
be able to take care of ourselves forever, so
our thoughts turn to long-term care and the

costs. Like I've said before, don't ignore your prognosis and don't ignore your finances. Get out ahead of things, so you can have as much control over your life now and in the future.

None of us can see into the future, so that made it hard to plan. What a challenge for me! I'm a planner and was used to making extensive plans for the whole year for both our city and for my life. Now I can't do that. But what I can do is ensure a safe and content future for myself.

You have to fully understand your financial position because that will inform your options. That's where my son was so helpful. He helped me understand my financial situation, and once I knew that, I could consider options. Please hear what I said: *I could consider options*. Not Howard, but me. I'm still in charge of my life; I don't put my head in the sand and avoid the truth.

> YOU HAVE TO FULLY UNDERSTAND YOUR FINANCIAL POSITION BECAUSE THAT WILL INFORM YOUR OPTIONS.

I refuse to avoid the truth and then let my life fall into Howard's lap. That's not productive, and it's not fair; in fact, it's selfish. I didn't want to be a burden to my family, and neither do you. So figure out your finances, then start making plans.

Right now—even today—start investigating how you'd like to be cared for while you still have the mental capacity to do it. Are you interested in and can afford a long-term living situation? Then start making appointments and taking tours now. There are countless facilities at various price points. Make a list of those that interest you and schedule a visit. If one place costs too much, check around. There are even non-profits that can help.

Find someone to guide you. Your doctor has connections, so start there. An attorney who knows elder care law is also a good resource.

If you have a house, can you sell it? Can you use your investments? Or Medicare? Social security? Life insurance?

Maybe you don't move into a long-term care facility but decide to have a paid caregiver in your home. Even with the federal government and Medicaid, you can pay a family member to be your caregiver. You have a lot of options, so check them all out.

Take care of yourself while you can. Otherwise, you'll lose all control over your life. You may be afraid and uncertain, but right now is your prime time. You won't be able to make decisions for yourself later, so get on with it!

Fear 5: I'm Grieving over Losing My Memory

I'm starting to stumble over words. I'll write something down, but when I go back and look at it, it doesn't look right to me. For example, the word *dog*. The words that used to look right to me no longer do. They just look different, and I second-guess myself. So later, I'll take a fresh look at the word in context to figure out if it's right.

When I look at someone, and we're talking, my brain and my mouth feel like they're not working together. So, I tend to look down as I concentrate rather than look them in the eye. This helps me focus on the point I'm trying to make, but I wonder if it's rude. I know how important it is to make eye contact, and I'm not able to do that like I did before. With the dementia, I have to concentrate more on what I am saying, and it's okay! This is how I cope with my condition.

I'm worried I won't recognize my family and when that will happen. No one knows. Even when in decline, you can remember people's voices, even though you may not always recognize faces. It's in and out. When it becomes permanent, I'll know it's closer to the end.

My friends and family are very important to my daily life. They're a piece of my life, and I don't want to lose them by forgetting their faces. I don't know if I'll feel the loss because I won't remember them. And that causes me grief now, while I still know them.

Losing my memory means I won't be able to write people notes anymore. I like to send cards to tell people I'm thinking about them. So what am I going to be able to do? If I can't read or write, what will I do?

> MY FRIENDS AND FAMILY ARE VERY IMPORTANT TO MY DAILY LIFE. THEY'RE A PIECE OF MY LIFE, AND I DON'T WANT TO LOSE THEM BY FORGETTING THEIR FACES.

I don't know what I'll be doing at that stage. I know that keeping your hands busy helps patients to cope, and they often knit or crochet. Movement is an important thing to help us keep going on a day-to-day basis.

As I'm driving to local things, I constantly say to myself, *Now where are you going?* I may have to remind myself four or five times before I get there. I say out loud, "I'm going to MidRivers Mall," or, "I'm going to Howard's." I have a conversation with myself to keep myself on track. Sometimes I can't remember where I'm going, so I remind myself.

The point is that I want to do what I want to do when I can. I don't know what tomorrow will bring, so I do everything I can and what I like today.

Fear 6: I'm Embarrassed about the Changes

Being embarrassed is a hot button for me. As a child, my mother controlled me by embarrassing me in front of other people. And it worked. It was like a weapon she used on me. Because of my childhood experiences, being embarrassed quickly flips to me feeling humiliated and blaming myself.

In my career, it didn't matter if I was a state rep, a county council member, or working a job. If someone embarrassed me, they were off my list. If I quit talking to you, it was very hard to get back in my graces. Once I cut you off, you were out. It was final. It was a burnt bridge, and I don't burn bridges.

But now, I'm afraid I might be the one embarrassing myself.

For example, in my professional career, I had to dress well, and I spent a lot of money on clothing. It was important to me to be my best and to act my best. But my ability to dress well has changed. It's shrunk.

There were four things I always paid careful attention to: my hair, my nails, my clothes, and my shoes. If I don't have one of them in place, I feel incomplete and slightly embarrassed. Keeping up with these things is costly;

> BUT NOW, I'M AFRAID I MIGHT BE THE ONE EMBARRASSING MYSELF.

I haven't bought clothes in two years because I'm on a fixed income. When my son helps with my budgeting, he always asks, "Is that important to you, Mom?" And yes, my appearance is important to me. It's what makes me feel like me. I'm embarrassed that I have to pick and choose what I can afford.

And I told you earlier how I've learned to manage my calendar. I struggle to be at the right place at the right time, and I'm embarrassed that I have to consult my calendar all the time. I have to check it two or three times because I get confused. I have to verify many times before I go to an appointment. That bothers me because I was once capable of checking my calendar at the beginning of the day, and I was off and running.

I'm fully cognizant that sometimes I get stuck. My mind doesn't always match my mouth, and after such an incident in public, someone once told me, "You shouldn't go out and speak in public the way you are acting." She thought I was embarrassing myself.

I thought, *Who are you to tell me not to do public speaking when you know I'm good at it and that's what I want to do?* At one time, this would have been a burn-the-bridge kind of comment. But I've known this woman for a long time, and it pushed me to think, *How can I get over this mouth and brain issue when I'm talking?*

So now, I'm sure to have notes. Even when I call someone on the phone, I first write down what I want to ask and why I'm calling. That helps me remember what I want to accomplish without wasting their time.

That helps me not get tongue-tied, and when I do, I laugh about it. I use humor to smooth things over.

Earlier, I mentioned that my way of telling someone I had early dementia was to engage them in conversation about what I'm doing now that I'm retired. I'd say I was writing a book about early dementia. For the first few times, nobody said a word after that. Nobody knew what to say, and the conversation died. That embarrassed me. I wanted to get the word out, but I had to live through several instances of this. It wasn't the fact of my dementia that embarrassed me, it was their response to that fact.

Sometimes I need a little time to process things, and I'm embarrassed when somebody gives me something to read, and I can't absorb it. The pressure of them waiting for me to comment embarrasses me. I can't handle that kind of pressure, so I had to figure out what to say in those situations.

> SOMETIMES I NEED A LITTLE TIME TO PROCESS THINGS . . .

At first, I panicked in these situations and had to figure out a coping mechanism. "Thanks for this. Let me read it and get back to you," I say. But when I get back to them, sometimes it's too late, and that's embarrassing.

Before, if you asked me a question, I knew the answer. Now I can't do that. I can't respond quickly or give my suggestions. My mind doesn't connect those dots anymore. I'm not what I used to be. I used to be quick, and I'm not anymore.

If you have someone in your life with dementia, choosing the right words is important in situations like these. If you say, "What's wrong with you?" it makes the person with dementia feel incompetent. It embarrasses them. Instead, say something like, "Why don't you get back to me when you can?" Extending grace goes a long way with me now.

Fear 7: I Don't Want to Be Isolated

My whole life has been about being with others, serving others, and enjoying others, and I don't ever want to be isolated. And that means I have to be proactive about reaching out. I can't sit around in my apartment waiting for someone to phone me, to invite me, or to include me. So like everything else, I get out ahead of it to make sure my calendar is full.

That means I'm constantly making plans for myself. I don't particularly like to phone people to make plans (of course, I'd rather they called me), but I do it anyway. Even though I don't like making phone calls, I do because it's necessary to stay in touch with the people I care about and who care about me. I don't wait around for them to call me because time goes by too fast, and I know they have busy lives. I'm not their top priority, but they like me and want to keep our relationship alive. So I take it on myself to reach out. Otherwise, I'd be very lonely.

> I DON'T WAIT AROUND FOR THEM TO CALL ME BECAUSE TIME GOES BY TOO FAST, AND I KNOW THEY HAVE BUSY LIVES.

Before I call, I look at my calendar to see what days I have open to meet. I ask them when it's good for them to have coffee, and we make plans from there. I have a purpose for each phone call and am ready to make a date with them.

I have some longtime friends from church who are important to me. Glenda has been my friend for fifty years, and I've been friends with Peggy and Nancy for close to forty years. We keep in touch at church and also at birthdays, and we help each other when needed.

I'm playing the piano at church again. I've always been part of the choir and have played the piano, and I've sung at church for many years. Now I play the piano every Sunday. We have Bible study on Wednesday nights.

These relationships are important to me because they've lasted for so long, and I want to maintain them. They've always included me, and I always include them, so I continue to reach out to them.

I also have political career friends through the places I've served. I try to keep in touch with people at each place where I served an elected position: Saint Charles Community College, Saint Charles County government, the Missouri House of Representatives, the city of Saint Charles. Since I don't see these people on a regular basis anymore, I get updates by reading the newspapers to keep up with state and local people. I see them at events and try to "work the room" to make sure I've spoken to everyone. I don't call these people because it's not appropriate. My plan for 2022 is to write them each a handwritten note and get out to a function once or twice to let them know I'm thinking about them. If I can help, I'm available.

Fifteen years ago, I joined a group I call FOF—Friends of Faith. These are a variety of women who work, give to the community, and serve on boards, and we keep in touch and get together periodically. In the summer, we have a pool party, and we schedule eating events and celebrate things at other people's houses. There's no specific rhythm to this group. Whenever someone wants to have a gathering, they send out an invitation to everyone with all the details. Sometimes I reach out and have one or another meet me for coffee.

My book club is also important to me, and we meet once a month at Bogey Hills Country Club. I don't always like the book that month, but we discuss it, and I say what I think. I can't wait to discuss this book with them!

For thirty-five years, I've been part of the Saint Charles Midday Rotary Club. I was one of the first five women members when the federal government mandated that they accept both men and women. In fact, I was the first woman president. We meet every Thursday, and we assist nonprofits by providing funds that make a difference in many lives. And it's another outlet of connection for me.

And then there's my eighth-grade graduation group consisting of four friends from Gundloch grammar school. A few years ago, we started to meet once a quarter for lunch, and we continue that today. Other than that, we keep in touch via Facebook.

People are important to me, so I keep reaching out. I keep showing up. I keep helping. I keep serving however I can, and I'm out of the house every day. My only local family is Howard, but I've made a huge family for myself.

> PEOPLE ARE IMPORTANT TO ME, SO I KEEP REACHING OUT. I KEEP SHOWING UP. I KEEP HELPING.

If this isn't your experience, it's never too late to make friends. There's always someone who wants to be heard and to connect. Here are some ways that you might reach out, even when you have early dementia.

- Volunteer. Someone needs your help. When you volunteer, you'll meet people who have similar interests.
- Say hello to strangers. Offer a positive comment.
- Join a book club.
- Join another type of club that revolves around something that interests you.
- Take lessons. Surely you can find something you'd like to know more about. Go to community classes, take private music or karate lessons. Keep moving and keep learning!

- Get on the computer. I look at my computer once a day, and I'm so glad I have it. No one else at my dinner table has one. I'm learning things as I'm going, and my computer keeps me alert. It's a big piece of staying aware and being connected to my life and friends and family. Even while I'm losing my memory, I'm learning new things. I think that helps my brain and strengthens it.

As you do these things, you'll meet people who like the same things you do, and you'll begin to build your circle, one person at a time.

4

A Son's Perspective on Caregiving

MY MOTHER WAS diagnosed with the early stages of dementia in 2020. When that happened, my life began changing from son to caregiver. Some of my first thoughts were, *How could this strong woman who raised me have dementia? How is she going to handle it? What changes are going to affect* my *lifestyle?*

My mother had always been a go-getter and in the mix of things. Her careers had been ones where she was always on the go and always outgoing. I didn't know how she would react to not being able to remember people, things, or events in her life. How would she react when people learned of her dementia?

I knew very little about dementia and had a lot to learn. I'm a planner and don't like anything unexpected.

I also knew my lifestyle was about to change. Before, my mother came over every

Sunday night to visit. It was usually for just an hour or so, and that was how we stayed in touch with her busy schedule. I realized rather quickly that our once-a-week visits wouldn't be enough. I'd need to check on her more often to make sure she was taking care of herself physically, mentally, and financially.

Mom had always been a private person regarding her financial affairs, as most of us are. I knew we'd need to discuss her finances regularly to make sure the bills were paid and to start planning for her later years. I'd also need to have access to her medical information (doctors, attorneys, contractors) in case something happened. I can't imagine anything more frustrating than having questions about her condition but not having access to the people who could answer them.

One of the first things I had her do was to start a notebook listing things like her doctors' contact information, the medicines she was taking, and the important things she felt I'd need to know in an emergency. I put them in a fire-proof safe in the house. We also started going through some of her belongings to see what was most important to her. We discussed which items she'd like to take with her when the time came for a memory facility and what that time would look like. One of the greatest gifts my mother gave to me was making her own decision to move into an independent living community that can transition to memory care. I didn't have to make that call; she did it for herself—and for me.

The advantage to having dementia, or any health issue, diagnosed early is that it gives people time to plan. People have time to gather information, to talk to others who've been through the same thing, and to consider options. It gives that person time to give input on decisions that will affect their final years.

Early diagnosis also gives the caregiver time to research what changes are coming and how to best handle them, rather than having to make quick decisions about how to best take care of their loved one. My mother and I have had time to take care of her finances, visit memory care units, and discuss how to tell family and friends about her dementia. Being able to do this made it easier to absorb what was happening and what steps needed to be taken as we traveled this path together.

We also started attending Alzheimer's group meetings at one of the local memory care facilities. These meetings were very help-ful because they provided answers to some of our questions or gave us direction regarding who to ask for answers. The other attendees were going through the same things and in varying stages. We could bounce our ideas off them and learn from their experiences.

One of the things I appreciate most about my experience with dementia is that it made me reevaluate my life plans and share them with my family at an early age instead of waiting. As stated before, I'm a planner, and having time to plan these things with my mother was a blessing in life instead of something I had to do alone.

—Howard Faith

5

In Closing

YES, WE HAVE dementia, and no, this isn't what we wanted—but that's okay. My life isn't over, and neither is yours, so don't give up! You are still valuable, you are still worthy, and you are still loved.

You may not have control over your dementia, but you do have control over your *attitude* about having dementia. Why not make it one of joy? Why not continue to spread good vibes? Why not grab on to everything you can to make these days happy and fulfilling?

That's what I'm trying to do. The things I've shared with you may not make you joyous. My goal is to share my ideas with you. Finding what works for you is what's important. Keep it simple, and don't give up. You may forget many things, but don't ever forget that living your life to the fullest is a choice you can make—even right now.

About the Author

Sally Faith was born in Fresno, California. She has been the director of Development for the Saint Charles Community College Foundation, director of Marketing for Whitmoor Country Club, and chair and vice chair of Saint Charles County Council, District 5. She's been a member of the

Saint Charles Transit Authority, Habitat for Humanity International, Athena Leadership Foundation, Saint Charles Rotary Club, and the Saint Charles and Saint Peters Chambers of Commerce. She's served on the board of directors of Bridgeway, Focus Saint Louis, Connections to Success, the New Frontier Bank, and Foundry Centre.

Sally was first elected to the Missouri House of Representatives in 2004. She was elected Mayor of Saint Charles, Missouri, in 2011, at which point she resigned her seat in the Missouri House of Representatives. She was reelected to a second term in April 2015.

Sally is happily situated in an independent living facility where she shares her apartment with her cats, Sweetie and Uno.

For every book sold, Sally is donating $1 to the Alzheimer's Association.